G000167068

BACK
FITNESS
THE YOGA WAY

The gentle, strengthening benefits of yoga are ideal for encouraging and maintaining a healthy back – whatever your age. Here are 26 yoga exercises, with many variations, to make your back strong, youthful and supple.

BACK FITNESS
THE YOGA WAY
Exercises and hints for a strong, supple back

by

KAREEN ZEBROFF

THORSONS PUBLISHERS LIMITED
Wellingborough, Northamptonshire

First published in the United Kingdom 1980

Original Canadian edition published by
Fforbez Publications Ltd, Vancouver, B.C.

© FFORBEZ PUBLICATIONS LIMITED 1979

British Library Cataloguing in Publication Data

Zebroff, Kareen
  Back fitness the yoga way.
  1. Back – Diseases
  2. Yoga, Hatha – Therapeutic use
  I. Title
  616.73 RM727

ISBN 0-7225-0685-6

Typeset by Ad'House, Earls Barton, Northampton
Printed in Great Britain by
Whitstable Litho Ltd., Whitstable, Kent

CONTENTS

Foreword

One of the first things developed after conception is the nervous system. This is the energizing force which generated your body and keeps on regenerating your cell structure. The nervous system is the life force which controls and co-ordinates all systems and functions of your body. This nervous system is housed and protected by the spine. Since every part of your body has a nerve supply and every nerve you have passes through small openings in the spine called 'foramina', it is of utmost importance to take proper care of your back.

Many people today have back problems which could be minimized if their muscles were better toned and their joints more agile. In this book Kareen Zebroff has covered the subject most thoroughly by first acquainting you with the function and anatomy of the spine. She then proceeds to explain how to cope with a back problem and, better still, how to prevent a back problem from occurring. Not only does she recommend numerous exercises for the back but she also prepares you for them, which is equally as important as the exercise itself. Keep in mind that certain exercises will always bother somebody, depending on their individual spine and the problem it might have. Any exercise causing pain should be stopped.

This book contains much information and many recommendations that chiropractors offer their patients daily. This is a book you will be proud to place on your book shelf for reliable information concerning the care of your spine. I believe that many people will find useful guidance here and that their health will benefit from it.

As a practising chiropractor I recommend *Back Fitness the Yoga Way* to anyone concerned about the future of their health and maintaining a happy, healthy feeling.

Elmer E. Raabe, D.C.

Introduction

Back Fitness the Yoga Way is for anyone who has ever suffered from a tired and aching back, who has been forced to groan and place a soothing hand on the small of the back after trying to straighten up in the garden, or who has experienced the painful spasms of tense back muscles. *It is not for people who suffer from severe disc-degeneration or other serious and chronic back problems.* For the proper diagnosis of your problem and if you have any doubts about exercising—consult your doctor or chiropractor.

In this book we are concerned with the ninety per cent of humanity who have a weak, a tense, a tired, and an aching back and who want to do something constructive about it. For you, we have good, sound advice to regain and maintain strength and muscle tone and to relax deep-seated tension. We want your spine to be strong and supple—in other words, youthful. We want you to get that spring back into your step, to move freely without worry over pain, to be able to laugh, dance and pursue sports with abandon.

Please pay particular attention to 'Prevention is the Best Cure' on page 21. Read it and reread it. It could be the most important part of the book for you.

1

Back Fitness the Yoga Way

It hurts too much to take out the kitchen rubbish; it will not let you straighten up after bending down for a while; it goes 'out' with every wrong move; it is our most common complaint: Bad Back.

The back is subject to terrific strain, which often results in injury. Designed to have the function of a suspension bridge, the spine has developed over the millenia into a fragile, delicately-balanced tentpole made up of twenty-nine building blocks. Many things can go wrong with it. Trauma may result from something as simple as the sudden jerking of an arm, a whiplash injury in a car accident, a bad fall, or a violent blow to the head and chin. Habitual misuse, such as lifting a heavy object without bending the legs or a gradual worsening of posture, is responsible for many back problems in later years.

If you already have a bad back, the chances are that it is also a weak one. Afraid of aggravating the bad condition, you will tend to favour the back and move it less freely than normal. The fear starts a vicious cycle: the worse the back is now, the stiffer and weaker you make it by limiting its movements. From there things go rapidly downhill—curvature (scoliosis) of the spine, slipped discs, low back pain, poor posture, poor breathing habits, back sprains, muscle spasms, osteoporosis, headaches, neuritis, inflammation and internal disorders may all follow.

The Yogis consider the spine the most important part of the anatomy because it houses and protects the spinal cord and spinal nerves, which lead from there to every part of the body. The nerves pass through tiny openings in the vertebrae, and if these are in any way distorted or not properly aligned, the nerves are pinched or irritated. This may result in pain down your legs or arms, numbness and tingling and eventual atrophy of the muscles.

For most of these ailments the gentle, strengthening exercises of yoga are greatly beneficial. Ask your doctor which of the exercises are best for your particular problem. But also consider consulting a chiropractor. Thoroughly schooled in all the basic sciences, his premise is that 'structure governs function'. He will analyze your spine thoroughly, particularly in respect to the nervous system. If there is any neural interference, abnormal cell structure development may be occurring in parts of the body served by the affected nerve.

Both chiropractors and doctors agree that exercise and good nutrition are prerequisites for a healthy back. Combine them with adequate rest, proper treatment, healthy mental attitude and good posture, and the healthful effects upon you should be miraculous.

In this book we will deal mainly with exercising your back to make it strong and supple—in other words, youthful. Yoga is the ideal method. Its slow movements and non-competitive aspects are suitable for anyone of any age or physical condition.

2

Knowing Your Back

Your back is made up of a spinal cord and a spinal column. The spinal cord is a column of nerve tissue which runs from your brain to your tail bone, receiving messages from nerve endings along the way and transmitting them back to the brain. The cord runs through protective bone called the spinal column, made up of twenty-nine small bones called vertebrae. Between the vertebrae are fluid-filled cushions of gristle called discs. The discs act as the shock absorbers of the spine.

Each vertebra is made up of several parts: a body which bears the weight, a process which forms the joints to which muscles attach themselves, and a canal, through which the spinal cord and nerves pass. This line of small bones, our spine, is in fact the supporter of the body, and virtually holds up the human frame.

The spine is divided into five distinct regions. The first, the *cervical* region, consists of the very flexible vertebrae of your neck and allows you to move your head freely from side to side, backward and forward.

The second, or *thoracic* region, is at the back of the chest area and is made up of less flexible but stronger vertebrae. They are attached to the ribs and the large muscles which allow you to lift heavy objects.

The third, or *lumbar* region, is generally known as the small of your back. This area is made up of five very strong bones which provide the flexibility for bending backwards, forwards and sideways freely.

The fourth, or *sacral* region, is found just above your buttocks. This bone is not very flexible because it is actually part of your pelvis and protects the reproductive organs, bladder and bowel.

The *coccyx*, or tailbone, is the lowest part of the spine. It is composed of five non-moveable segments. Because they have been fused together, they are strong and able to withstand a great deal of strain.

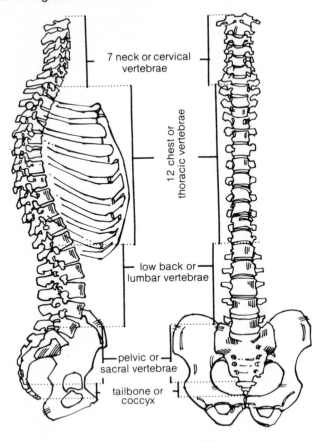

7 neck or cervical vertebrae

12 chest or thoracic vertebrae

low back or lumbar vertebrae

pelvic or sacral vertebrae

tailbone or coccyx

Fig. 1a. Human spine, side view and back view.

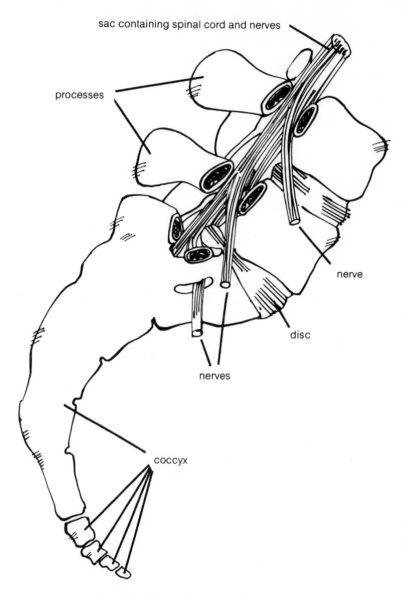

Fig. 1b. Disc, spinal cord and coccyx.

3

Common Back Problems

Many things can go wrong with the back. The two most common problems are:
- — Slipped disc, which occurs most often in the lumbar and cervical regions of the back. It can cause severe pain because the outer ring of cartilage has lost its supportive power and the soft jelly-like centre bulges out from between the vertebrae and rubs against the spinal nerve.
- — Scoliosis, can be common to all ages, but usually originates in childhood. A spinal curvature develops because of the body's effort to keep the head in balance over the tailbone.

Other problems are:
- — Arthritis, when joints of the back become inflamed.
- — Osteoporosis, where increasing porosity and a thinning of the bones of the spine causes much pain. It is also responsible for loss of height, and a bent-over appearance.
- — Lordosis, an exaggerated arch in the lower back is often caused by poor posture.
- — Ligament and tendon strain and tear, which is a result of sudden movement or of forcing the spine beyond its point of flexibility.

— Degenerate disc occurs when the discs start to break down and disintegrate gradually.
— A bad back results in various curvatures and misaligned vertebrae. This will result in improper nerve energy to various organs and other parts of the body and may impair their function.

4

Nutrition for Your Back

Even your back needs good nutrition. In fact, an adequate supply of vitamin C and protein are a daily must for good *development* of the bone. Calcium, vitamin D, phosphorus, magnesium and essential trace minerals are necessary for *maintaining* good skeletal health; without them, demineralization of the bones can occur. But calcium also delays fatigue by helping to maintain muscle tone, strong muscular contraction and good posture. If calcium is taken about an hour before strenuous exercise, it will help to prevent muscle cramp and spasm. Calcium gluconate, by the way, is an excellent painkiller when injected directly into your veins by your doctor. It is interesting that, by studying control groups of women in which half suffered from osteoporosis and half did not, scientists found that healthy women consumed an average of 862mg of calcium and 76.6g of protein daily, whereas the afflicted women averaged only 584mg of calcium and 61g of protein.

Many backaches are caused by the inability of the spine to put up with tension arising from emotional stress. This will manifest itself in the form of knotted muscles in the neck, shoulders and lower back. Many health authorities agree that pain from tension can be relieved through proper rest, relaxing yoga exercises and such natural, nutritional relaxers in your diet as:
— calcium in milk

- leafy greens
- molasses
- phosphorus in protein foods such as meat and dairy products
- 1-2 tablespoonsful cold-pressed vegetable oils daily
- vitamin D from sunshine and sunlamps
- cod-liver oil
- wholewheat, brown rice
- lecithin
- the B-vitamin complex, particularly B_1, B_2, and B_6, as found in brewer's yeast, molasses, grains, vegetables and nuts.

5

Prevention is the Best Cure

Few people appreciate their good health until something goes wrong. Then they ask, 'Why?' and 'Why me?' There are many reasons, of course. Incorrect posture—the way you sit, stand and sleep—is just one example of what can contribute to a bad back.

Interestingly enough, many yoga teachers started their yoga studies because of back problems. They may never be able to do certain advanced poses, but they have improved their general health tremendously and because they have exercised and strengthened the back, their symptoms have abated.

After consulting doctors, chiropractors, books and people who have had bad backs in the past, I have come up with the following advice for a healthy back:

1. Avoid standing for long periods of time. It builds up pressure on the small of your back.

2. If you must stand for some time, put your foot up on a low stool and lean with your elbow on the bent knee. This straightens the small of the back.

3. Sleep on a firm mattress. Avoid sleeping on your stomach. If you sleep on your back, have your head on a pillow and another under your knees. It is best to lie on your side, with your knees slightly flexed.

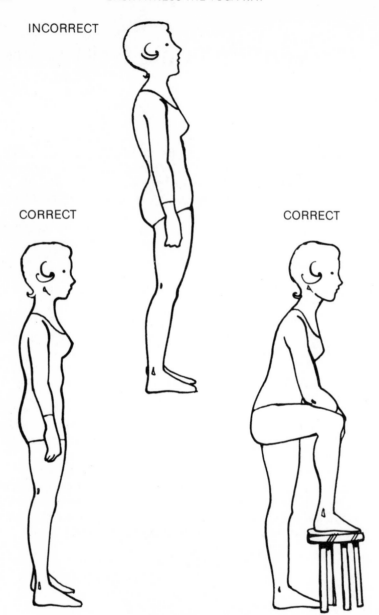

Fig. 2. Standing postures.

INCORRECT   CORRECT

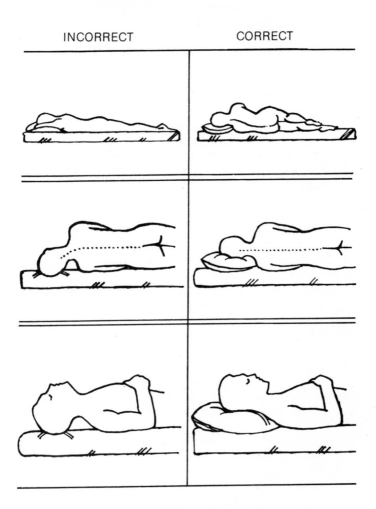

Fig. 3. Sleeping positions.

4.   Even the way you get up in the morning is important. Turn on your side and swing your legs off the bed, then push yourself into a sitting position with your arms. This will minimize the amount of strain on the back.

5.   Do not watch TV in bed with your head propped at a sharp angle.

6.   Always lift heavy objects with knees bent, to avoid straining and tearing of muscles, ligaments and tendons of the back. (See Figure 4 for proper lifting techniques.)

7.   Cross your legs at the ankles only. Crossing at the knee aggravates existing back conditions and cuts off circulation in the lower limbs, causing varicose veins, spider veins and swollen ankles.

8.   Always sit in a firm, straight-backed chair. Avoid fat, over-stuffed chairs and sofas.

9.   Never push yourself beyond your abilities. Know your own physical limitations and build up strength gradually.

10. Go on a diet. The extra weight you carry around puts stress on the back, legs and heart.

11. Exercise. If you are sitting most of the day, get up and move about during coffee breaks. Try to get in a late-at-night or early-morning walk or gentle yoga workout—even if it is only for ten minutes. Learn to fidget, to adjust your position often.

12. Tilt, tilt, tilt! Tilting the pelvis forward (models call it tucking) straightens the small of the back and strengthens the muscles of both the buttocks and the abdomen. It relieves low backache, and is the best and most attractive way to walk.

INCORRECT

CORRECT

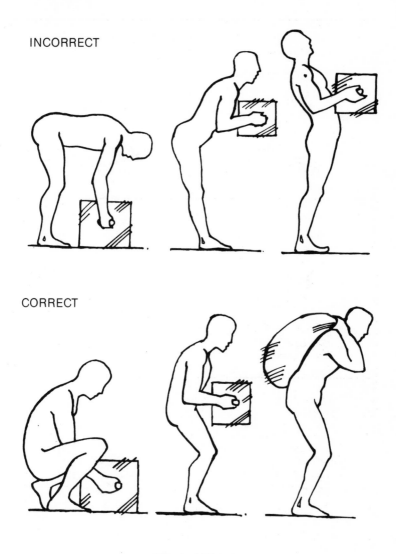

Fig. 4. Lifting.

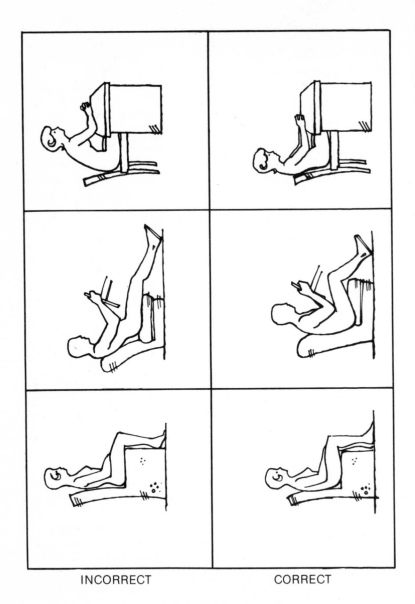

INCORRECT   CORRECT

Fig. 5. Sitting positions.

13. Tighten the stomach muscles, pinch the buttocks together, tilt the pelvis forward and *exhale* every time you want to lift something, carry something or pull your legs up.

14. Move *slowly* in and out of exercises or positions that give you pain or stiffness.

15. Unless you have varicose veins, learn to squat often to strengthen the leg muscles and the pelvis.

16. Put one foot on a low stool, whenever you have to bend forward from the waist (looking after a baby, brushing your teeth, washing dishes).

17. Never lock your knees in. Keep the knees slightly flexed or bent.

18. Keep warm at all times, to prevent the muscles from getting stiff and tense. Have a warm bath, wear warm clothing, use a warm hot water bottle wrapped in towelling, invest in an electric blanket.

19. Your next big present should be a rocking-chair— even if you have to give it to yourself. The gentle rocking action improves circulation and keeps the spine mobile. It is best with a foot-stool.

20. Place a foot-stool in front of the toilet, too. You may find it most comfortable to put only one foot on it.

21. Wear low-heeled shoes with soft, thick soles and lots of toe-room. High heels cause painful jarring, loss of balance and poor posture.

22. Avoid the constant use of girdles. It gives false security and encourages weak muscles. Instead, gently strengthen the back through exercise, frequent moving and walks.

23. Do not ignore pain-signals. Rest in the sleeping position (Figure 3), stretch slowly, apply heat and consult your doctor or chiropractor.

24. When you suffer from back pain, avoid car-riding unless you can lie down in the back seat, avoid long flights and straight chairs. If you must sit, place a pillow behind your buttocks.

25. To support you during a sneeze, laugh or cough, and to prevent you from being thrown forward uncontrollably, tighten your stomach muscles, cross your hands and press them against your belly.

26. For women only: many backaches are gynaecological in nature. Check with your doctor. Tampons often cause backache so switching to sanitary towels may bring relief.

27. Do not lean against walls or against counters with your hip. Avoid propping babies or groceries against your hips. The shoulders are the best place for carrying. Remember, to keep your spine straight you must tilt the pelvis forward. Ideally, you should stand with knees slightly bent, feet slightly outward and chest lifted. Breathe deeply, keep your head and chin up, keep your shoulders down, tighten your stomach, tuck buttocks under and walk softly!

6

Rules of Yoga Practice

1. *Never compare yourself to anyone else.* Yoga emphasizes personal progress. Be careful not to go beyond the limit of your capability. By performing the exercise regularly you are bound to do better today than you did yesterday. In yoga there is visible progress. You will find that after a relatively short time you will be able to get into more advanced poses without any danger of strain.

2. *Never hurry.* Go into the postures *slowly,* taking ten to fifteen seconds to get from the beginning to the holding position. This gives bonus benefits, makes each exercise more effective and prevents injury.

3. *Hold each position* after you have gone as far into it as comfort permits. Muscles must undergo sustained effort in order to stay in condition. As a beginner, hold each posture at its extremity for five seconds. Increase this time by five seconds a week as you improve. Through the holding position you are doing an exercise over and over, as it were, and therefore an exercise need be repeated only three times, instead of twenty.

4. *Breathe normally* during the holding position of an exercise. There is a tendency for most people to hold their breath while they desperately and tensely hold on. This is

absolutely wrong. Yoga stresses relaxation, even while exercising. You should go as far into a pose as comfort permits, then relax there and breathe as normally as comfort permits. As a student advances in proficiency, there is a prescribed way of breathing with each exercise. Generally speaking, one should exhale when going into a pose and inhale as one comes out of it. The notable exceptions are the Cobra and the Locust.

5. *Never force a position.* Never jerk or bounce in order to 'go further'. Go as far as you can, then hold it there. Pain is a danger signal devised by the body to stop immediately or risk injury. If, as in calisthenics, you are moving so fast that your momentum does not permit you to stop short, you can easily move past the danger signal and get hurt. This is what has happened when you experience muscular soreness or muscle strain.

6. *Concentrate intensely* with each exercise you perform. This is especially necessary in balancing exercises. Avoid moving your head rapidly, speaking or laughing self-consciously when you exercise. Visualizing encourages concentration which, in turn, promotes quality of action. For instance, pretend to be a fierce lion in the Lion or a pussy-cat just up from her nap in the Cat Stretch. It will make exercising more fun and improve concentration.

7. *Come out of an exercise as slowly* as you went into it. Not only do you lose at least a third of the value if you permit yourself to collapse, but you might even risk injury.

8. *Rest between exercises.* The beauty of yoga lies in its gentleness. You need never experience draining fatigue or painful, sore muscles. Catch your breath, let the muscles rebound from a delightful stretch and permit the body to assimilate what it has learned.

9. *Always keep your body relaxed,* even at the apex of a position, except for those parts which are directly involved in the pose. For example, in the Cobra concentrate on the back

and keep the buttocks and thighs relaxed. The effort you are making should never be mirrored in a distorted face.

10. *The best time* to exercise is either first thing in the morning or last thing at night. You may prefer a short period at each of these times; it depends on your particular need. In the morning the body is still stiff, but the exercises will help you to work better all day. In the evening the exercising comes more easily and refreshes and relaxes you for a good sleep. Learn to use exercises as energizers or relaxers throughout the day.

11. *Practise regularly,* even if you have time for only a few exercises on some days. Then, do only those poses that you know do *you* the most good. Make yoga as integral to your daily routine as eating and sleeping. You will notice that the new strength and flexibility of your spine will give you welcome relief from your chronic backache.

12. *Good posture* usually means good health. Strive to maintain your body in its normal position. Military standards for good posture may help you to improve yours.

7

Exercise Schedules

Your back can become stiff and painful in a very short time if you do not exercise it. Inactivity of the muscles may cause them to shrink and become taut, thus limiting the extent of your movement. Therefore it is essential that you use and *stretch these muscles to keep your back supple.* Always check with your doctor or chiropractor which exercises are suitable and safe for you.

Exercises to Rejuvenate Stiff Muscles
Alternate Leg Stretch
Crossbeam
Camel
Spread Leg Stretch
Cobra
Shoulder-stand
Crossed Knee Bend
Leg-over

Exercises to Strengthen the Back Muscles
Pendulum
Sit-up
Spread Leg Stretch

Exercises for Keeping the Sacroiliac, Lumbar and Dorsal Area Healthy
Boat
Rock 'n' Rolls
Crossbeam
Reverse Arch
Crossed Knee Bend
Cobra

Exercises to Relax Tension
Bow
Knee Press
Twist
Alternate Leg Stretch
Deep Lunge

For Arthritis in the Back
Blade
Pendulum

For Sciatic Pain
Half Shoulder-stand
Knee and Thigh Stretch
Spread Leg Stretch

For Relief of Severe Back Pain
Staff
Reverse Arch
Crossed Knee Bend (lower back)

For the Injured Back and Correction of Posture and Whiplash
Blade
Bow
Camel
Leg-over
Staff

Exercises for Slipped Discs

Boat
Locust
Bow
Cobra

Realignment of Vertebrae

Cobra
Twist

$(Rajeev + Girgi)^2 = (\qquad)^4$

Castle Gate.

Locust and I face you always will

Mrs Geeta Rowlley

Daniel S. Eastley. 8.30 8.30

85 12

Realignment after stretch Rowlley 13.00 3½
Daniel Daniel Rowlley 14.00
Realignment 10.00 15.00 hours.
Real lley 11.00 16.00
8.30 4.30 5.30 12.00 16.30.

1 2 3 4 5 6 7 8 9 10.

1.00
10.50 Slipped disc Geeta Nath. Slipped Discs
10.50 10.50 1 2 3 4 5 Slipped Discs
Realign 10.50 1 2 3 4 5 Geeta Nath.
10.50 Locust Geeta Nath.

Boat Torust G Geeta Nath Geeta Nath
Geeta Nath
Geeta Nath
Exercise for Slipped Discs Slipped Discs
Boat Geeta Nath. Geeta Nath Geeta Nath.
Locust Boat Locust Geeta Nath. Geeta Nath
Realignment. Boat Locust. Geeta Nath
Geeta Nath. Boat Locust. Geeta Nath
R Geeta Nath. Geeta Nath. Geeta Nath
Geeta Nath.
7.50 Geeta Nath.
7.50 Geeta Nath.
7.52.

D Coxen
A Coxen

8

Yoga Exercises

Therapeutic Poses for the Bad Back
All the yoga poses in this book are gentle enough for your back if done slowly and if the number of repetitions is increased gradually over a number of weeks. But, for the 'bad' back, chiropractors and therapists specifically recommend the following little exercises (in which your surroundings *assist* you till you are stronger) and familiar yoga poses.

 Boat Variations
 Bow Variation I
 Sit-Up Variations
 Arm & Leg Stretch (tummy against the wall)
 Pendulum
 Cat Stretch Variations
 Rock 'n' Rolls
 Reverse Arch
 Deep Lunge
 Knee Press

ALTERNATE LEG STRETCH

Benefits
 — Strengthens back muscles.
 — Reduces tension from the legs, buttocks and back.

— Massages most abdominal organs and stimulates them into action.
— Rejuvenates by making the spine supple and strong.

Technique
1. Sit on the floor, legs stretched out, back straight.
2. Bend your left leg and, keeping the side of the knee on the floor, bring your left foot against the right thigh, close to the body (Figure 6a).
3. Stretching the arms out, slide them SLOWLY down your leg as far as you can reach, bending forward with a curling motion of the spine (Figure 6b).
4. Grasp the leg; this may be at the knee, calf or ankle, depending on your flexibility.
5. Bend the elbows out and down, and gently pull yourself forward and down. Avoid strain by making this a smooth, not jerky, motion.
6. Go only as far as you comfortably can and then hold the position 5-30 seconds. Breathe normally (Figure 6c).
7. Straighten up slowly and repeat on the other side.
8. Perform three times on each side.

Dos and Don'ts
— It is amazing how quickly, with perseverance, you will be able to bring your head to your knee. A stiff spine and tense hamstring muscles are one of the first indications of age. This asana will loosen both areas in even the most inflexible.
— DON'T bend your knees and refrain from jerking. It is the motionless holding of the yoga positions that does the most effective work and prevents strain.

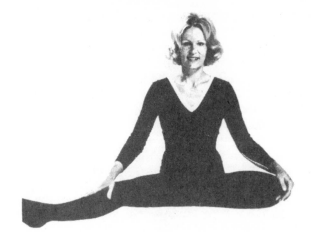

Fig. 6a

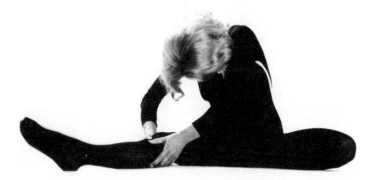

Fig. 6b

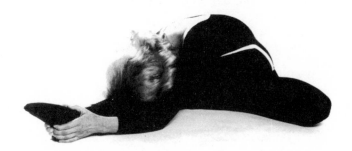

Fig. 6c

ARM AND LEG STRETCH

Benefits
— Strengthens and relieves pain in the lower back.
— Promotes grace and poise through improved balance.
— Relieves tension of the back and thighs.
— Gives a most pleasant massage to vertebrae through the gentle backward stretch.

Technique
1. Stand straight, heels together, toes slightly pointed outward.
2. Raise your arm slowly so that it stands out at an angle but the hand is above the head. The elbows are straight.
3. Bend your left leg at the knee, bringing it close to the buttocks, and shift your body weight onto the right foot.
4. Grasp your left foot with your left hand (Figure 7a).
5. Bend backward from the waist, at the same time pulling on the foot and moving the right arm as far back as balancing permits. Let the head drop back (Figure 7b).
6. Hold this position for five seconds at the start, increasing the time at five seconds a week.
7. Repeat on the other side and perform the asana three times on each side.

Variation
1. As above, but facing and barely touching a wall.
2. Bend one knee, grasp the ankle and pull it against the buttock.
3. Hold, relax. Repeat on other side.

Dos and Don'ts
— DO simple balancing exercises such as the Tree first, if you have difficulty keeping your balance.
— DO concentrate fiercely, it will help you to keep your balance better.
— DO move slowly when going into and coming out of the Arm and Leg Stretch, as in all yoga exercises.
— DON'T close your eyes.

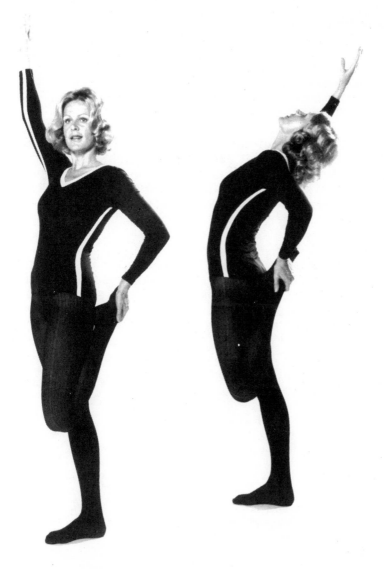

Fig. 7a   Fig. 7b

BLADE

Benefits
— Relieves bursitis and arthritic pain.
— Relieves tension in shoulders and upper back.

Technique
1. Sit in a comfortably cross-legged position.
2. Bend your elbows and bring them up at the sides, fingertips touching in front of your chest (Figure 8a).
3. Draw the shoulder blades together as though you had to hold onto a £1 note between them. Keep elbows up as much as possible.
4. Hold the pose for 5-10 seconds (Figure 8b).
5. Release the pose slowly. Shrug your shoulders.
6. Repeat 3-5 times.

Dos and Don'ts
— DO relax momentarily tense muscles by shrugging them. The shoulders are usually the first seat of tension and may, at first, complain about being stretched out of their cramped position.
— DON'T raise your shoulders as you pinch them and try to keep the elbows up.

Sit in a comfortably comfortably.

$1 + 1 = 2$

$2 + 4 = 6$

$7\frac{1}{2}$

$7.\frac{1}{2}$

$7.\frac{1}{2}$ -

$7\frac{1}{2}$

5

35

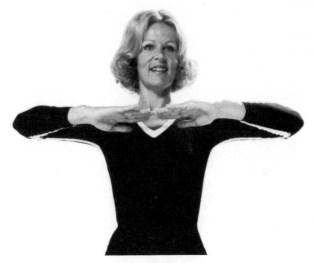

Fig. 8a

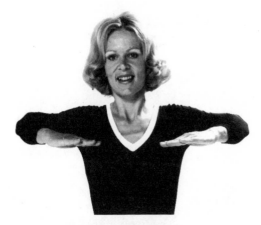

Fig. 8b

THE BOAT

Benefits
— Is beneficial to people with a slipped disc.
— Stretches and limbers up the spine.
— Relieves pain in the sacral and lumbar areas of the back.

Basic Technique
1. Lie on your stomach on the floor, arms stretched back, face down (Figure 9a).
2. All at the same time, slowly lift your head, chest and legs as far as they will go.
3. Lift your arms a few inches off the floor but parallel to it.
4. Pinch your buttocks together and keep the legs stretched straight and together (Figure 9b).
5. Hold, breathing normally, for as long as you can, or 5-30 seconds.
6. Repeat twice more.

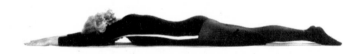

Fig. 9a

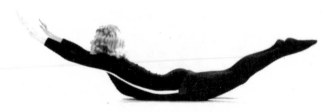

Fig. 9b

Variation 1
For people whose doctor or chiropractor says that they may
not bend backward.
   1. With a firm rolled blanket (or sleeping bag tightly rolled)
      under your hips, anchor your feet under a couch.
   2. With your hands by your side, slowly raise your upper
      body so it is in a straight line with your legs. Do not
      arch backwards (Figure 9c).
   3. Hold, relax, repeat.
   4. Turn yourself around so that you are now grabbing the
      legs of the couch with both your hands. The firm roll
      should be under your *waist* (Figure 9d).
   5. Slowly raise both legs together, hold, lower, relax.
      Repeat.

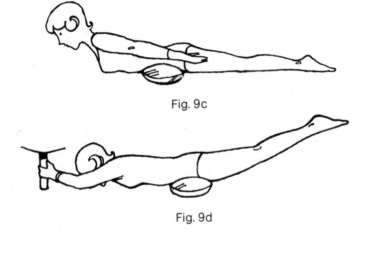

Fig. 9c

Fig. 9d

Fig. 9e

Variation 2
1. Lie on the floor, arms outstretched or folded under your head (Figure 9e).
2. Tighten buttocks. Hold, relax. Repeat several times.

Variation 3
1. Lie on the floor, arms outstretched and heels under a couch or chair (Figure 9f).
2. Lift your arms and upper body slowly. Relax. Repeat twice.

Variation 4
1. As above, but put a firm roll under your hips.
2. Lift your left arm and shoulder, hold, lower, relax. Repeat on the other side (Figure 9g).

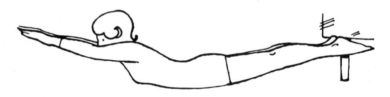

Fig. 9f

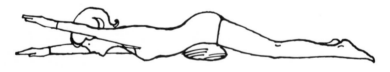

Fig. 9g

Variation 5
1. Put a firm roll under your waist.
2. Fold arms under your head, raise right leg. Hold, lower, relax. Repeat with other leg (Figure 9h).

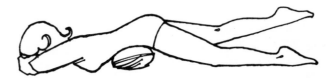

Fig. 9h

Dos and Don'ts
— DO make sure that your legs are together for greater benefit.
— DON'T let the hands support you, for a good work-out of the muscles of the upper back.
— DON'T give up if your legs and chest will not lift too far off the floor at first. This will come.

The Boat is a gentler version of the more advanced Locust but has more of its benefits without the strain. For the elderly, or people with back problems, the Boat is safe and effective because you are working against gravity and therefore can never go too far.

BOW

Benefits
— Relieves pain from a slipped disc.
— Tones and firms the muscles of the abdomen, arms, legs and back.
— Strengthens and limbers up the spine.
— Improves posture.
— Relieves pain and strengthens lower back.

Technique
1. Lie face down on your abdomen, hands by your side.
2. Bend your knees and bring them close to your buttocks.
3. Grasp your legs at the ankles, one at a time (Figure 10a).
4. Lift your knees off the floor by pulling the ankles *away* from the hands. You will still be tightly holding on, but it is the *away* motion rather than a *down* pull that will do the trick.
5. Lift your head at the same time (Figure 10b).
6. Hold the position for 5-10 seconds at the first, increasing to 30 seconds at 5 seconds a week. Breathe normally.
7. Slowly relax and rest for awhile.
8. Repeat twice more.

Variation
1. As above.
2. Bend one knee, grasp the ankle and pull it towards the buttock. Leave head down.
3. Hold. Relax. Repeat with other leg.

Dos and Don'ts
— DO come out of the exercise slowly.
— DO pull the ankles 'up and away' rather than down to get those stubborn knees off the ground.
— DON'T collapse in a heap. You will get more exercise for your time.

This is a demanding but most beneficial exercise and should be included in your schedule.

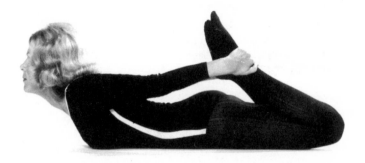

Fig. 10a

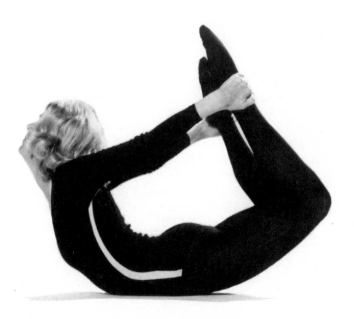

Fig. 10b

CAMEL

Benefits
— Makes the spine flexible and tones it.
— Improves posture.
— Benefits rounded shoulders, hunched backs.
— Beneficial to the elderly or people with spinal injuries, because it is so gentle.

Technique
1. Kneel in an upright position, keeping the legs together, toes pointed back.
2. Place hands on the waist and bend slowly backward, pushing the pelvis forward (Figure 11a).
3. Let the head hang back.
4. Let the right hand hang down over the heel, then the left (Figure 11b), and put palms on the feet, if possible.
5. Pinch the buttocks together, pushing the thighs and pelvis well forward (Figure 11c).
6. Hold this position for as long as possible or from 5-30 seconds. Breathe normally.
7. Repeat twice more.

Dos and Don'ts
— DO remember to keep the chest and pelvis thrust forward for a better bend.
— DON'T press beyond a point of comfort.

At first your hands will only hang slackly down in mid-air and as a beginner you needn't worry about touching your feet. This asana is so gentle and yet gives such an effective stretch to the spine, that anyone over middle age can safely practise it.

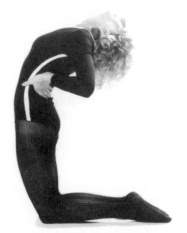

Fig. 11a

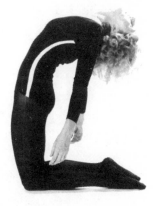

Fig. 11b

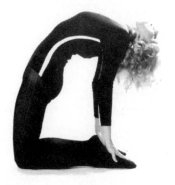

Fig. 11c

CAT STRETCH

Benefits
— Strengthens the back.
— Reduces tension.
— Relieves pain in lower back.

Technique: Cat Rock
1. Kneel on all fours.
2. Arch the upper back up, tightening the buttocks and pulling the head between the arms. Keep your elbows straight (Figure 12a).
3. Now squeeze your back down, bring your head up and stick bottom out.
4. Slowly rock up, down, up, down.

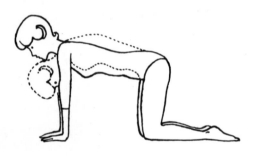

Fig. 12a

Technique: Cat Stretch
1. Kneel on all fours.
2. Rocking slightly back first, (Figure 12b) lower your chest in a sweeping motion, trying to rest the Adam's apple on the floor (Figure 12c).
3. Hold the position for 5 seconds, with most of the weight on the arms.
4. Return to the first position and arch the back in an upward motion rather like an angry, spitting cat (Figure 12d).

5. Hold for 5 seconds, relax.
6. Now bring your right knee towards the head, and touch it if you can. Hold 5 seconds (Figure 12e).
7. Stretch the leg out and up in back, keeping it straight. Hold. Keep the head up and arms straight (Figure 12f).
8. Return the leg slowly to the head. Hold.
9. Relax. Repeat on the other side.
10. Repeat the whole series once more.

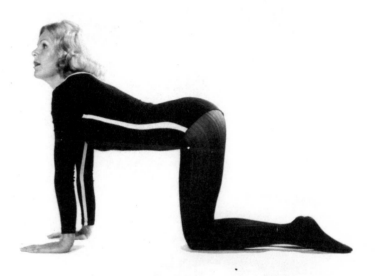

Fig. 12b

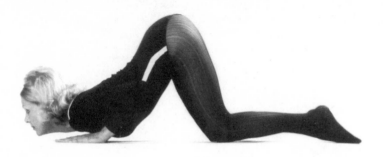

Fig. 12c

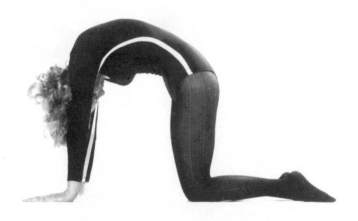

Fig. 12d

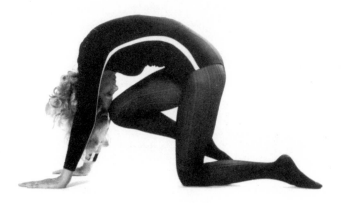

Fig. 12e

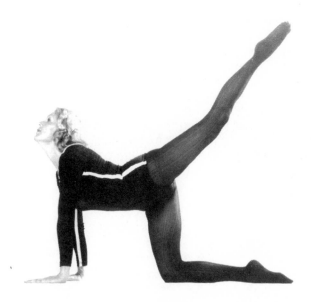

Fig. 12f

Variation 1

1. Kneel on all fours.
2. Raise your right arm and stretch it towards the ceiling as though to touch it. Hold.
3. Bring right arm up, stretch and look at it. Hold.
4. Repeat both poses several times.

Dos and Don'ts

— DO enjoy the stretching movement of your body. Move slowly and with grace.
— DON'T be discouraged by not getting your knees to your head for a while. It will come.

The Cat Stretch is a particularly fine exercise for relaxing. It is recommended by gynaecologists after childbirth and helps with those vague aches and pains in the lower back and abdominal area.

CHAIR HULA

Benefits

— Strengthens backs, hip and thigh muscles.
— Relieves tense and painful back.
— Stretches spine and extends discs.

Technique

1. Grip back of chair, hands well apart.
2. Do hula by first moving hips to the right, to the back, to the left and then tilting the pelvis forward.
3. With knees slightly bent, describe big circles smoothly, feeling the pull of muscles in the back, hips and thighs.
4. Repeat 15-30 times, describing circles to the left also.

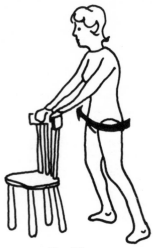

Fig. 13a

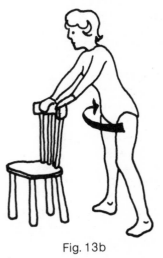

Fig. 13b

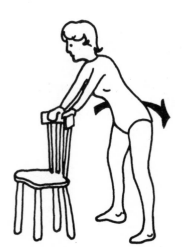

Fig. 13c

COBRA

Benefits

— Stretches and realigns the vertebrae of the spinal column. (Beneficial for people with a slipped disc.)
— Strengthens the abdomen and muscles of the back.

Technique
1. Lie on your stomach, hands by your side, feet together.
2. Bring the hands, palms down, under the shoulders, a shoulder's width apart (Figure 14a).
3. Lift your head SLOWLY, looking up at the ceiling.
4. When the head is up as far as it will go, and only then, lift the upper shoulders and back, making the muscles of the back do most of the work, rather than the hands.
5. Continue lifting the trunk until you can go no further and still keep the pubic area on the floor. There should be a good arch in the lower spine, but the arms need not be straight (Figure 14b).
6. Hold this position for as long as is comfortable (5-30 seconds).
7. Slowly come out of the Cobra position, feeling the action of each vertebra rolling against the next, and leaving your head up to the very last.
8. Repeat twice more; breathe normally while holding.

Dos and Don'ts
— DO make sure that your eyes look upward in their sockets throughout going into, holding and coming out of the exercise. Be aware of and enjoy the slow movement of your spine, the vertebra-by-vertebra massage.

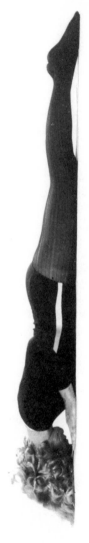

Fig. 14a

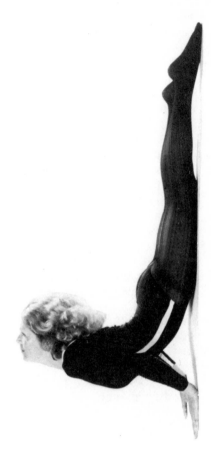

Fig. 14b

CROSSBEAM

Benefits
— Flattens the abdominal region.
— Tones and firms the inner thigh.
— Relieves stiff backs.
— Stretches the entire pelvic area.
— Stimulates the abdominal organs.

Technique
1. Kneel in an upright position on the floor keeping the feet together.
2. Stretch your right leg out to the right, keeping the knee straight and the toes pointed to the front.
3. Lift both arms out to the side (Figure 15a).
4. Place your right arm onto the right leg, palm up.
5. Bend your body to the right, resting the right ear on the arm (Figure 15b).
6. Lift the left arm slowly over the head, eventually bringing it straight over the right hand, palms touching.
7. Keep your face forward, so that you are peeking through the opening created by the arms (Figure 15c).
8. Hold for a comfortable period (5-30 seconds), breathing normally throughout.

Dos and Don'ts
— DON'T get discouraged if you are nowhere near the ideal at first. One of the amazing qualities of yoga is how fast you can improve.
— DON'T bend forward from the waist, but make it a sideways stretch.

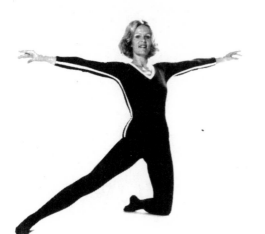

Fig. 15a

Fig. 15b

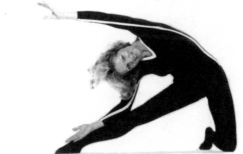

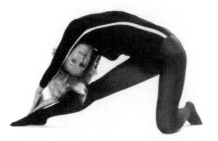

Fig. 15c

CROSSED KNEE BEND

Benefits
— Relieves morning backache.
— Is excellent for sacroiliac troubles.
— Is a good breathing exercise in its own right.

Technique
1. Stand, with the spine erect.
2. Cross the right knee over the left one and keep it slightly bent. Place the toes beside each other, but keep the heel up.
3. Inhale deeply, then bend slowly forward while exhaling, keeping the spine centred, the shoulders straight.
4. Try to touch the fingers to the floor or as far as you can. Relax, letting the head hang loosely (Figure 16).
5. Now make sure that you have *exhaled completely,* then deliberately *relax* the abdomen. A few seconds will pass, then the abdomen will slowly be sucked in by the vacuum you have created by exhaling.
6. Straighten up gradually and inhale.
7. Repeat three times with each leg.

Variation
As above but keep head up.

Dos and Don'ts
— DO use a low stool or hassock, at first, to give you confidence.
— DO keep the spine centred throughout the pose. Avoid the tendency to push a hip to the side.
— DON'T round the shoulders and bend the hips; bend from the waist only.
— DO persist, if the stomach does not want to be sucked in at first. You are either, a) not relaxing it, b) have not exhaled completely, or c) are not waiting the few seconds of complete relaxation it takes to have this fascinating phenomenon happen.

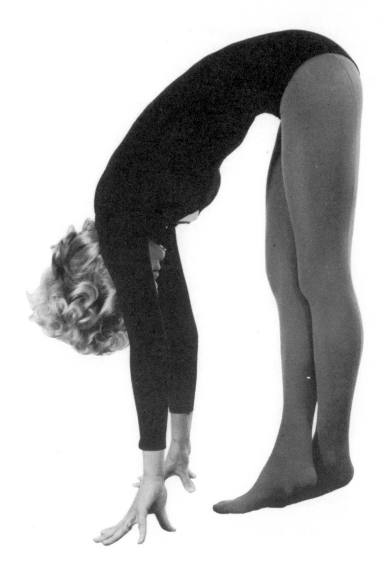

Fig. 16

DEEP LUNGE

Benefits
— Strengthens and firms the thighs and calves.
— Promotes balance and thereby poise.
— Relaxes the tension in the back.
— Stretches hip flexors.

Technique
1. Stand, the feet about 30 ins apart.
2. Turn the right foot to a 90° angle to the body, the left foot pointing straight forward.
3. Bend your right knee and shift the body weight onto the right leg.
4. EXHALE, clasp your hands behind your back and bend the body forward, resting the chest on the right thigh (Figure 17a).
5. At the same time, slide the left leg back as far as possible, keeping the knee straight. Hold. Straighten up. Relax. Or, for the more advanced:
6. Having established your balance, now slowly slide the chest off the thigh on the inside and attempt to bring the forehead to the floor.
7. Hold for 10-30 seconds, breathing normally (Figure 17b).
8. EXHALE, straighten up slowly and relax.
9. Repeat on the other side. Repeat on both sides twice more.

Dos and Don'ts
— DO keep the left foot pointed forward to give you a broader base of balance.
— DO use the hands as support at the beginning.
— DO use your body weight to help you bring the head closer to the floor, rather than jerking or forcing.
— DON'T bend your left knee.

The Deep Lunge combines many benefits for the whole leg and is particularly recommended for athletes and for ladies who want the firm look and a supple spine.

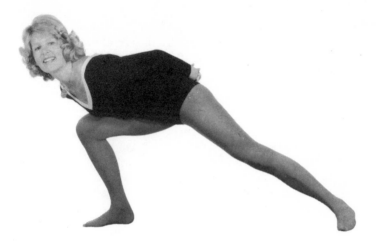

Fig. 17a

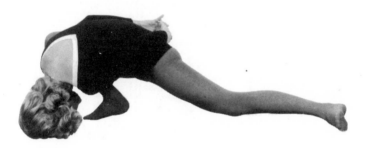

Fig. 17b

DOOR HANG

The door hang puts you 'into traction' at home. That is, it helps to relieve pressure by the discs on the sciatic nerve and aligns the spine, permitting the discs to slip back into their natural position. It improves posture.

Technique
1. Place a folded towel over the top of the open door.
2. Place hands over towel and door and bend your knees parallel to the floor. Relax and let yourself hang free.
3. Now, deliberately let your lower back and pelvis drop. You are stretching your back, rather than the arms.
4. Hang as long as comfort permits. Stand up, relax a few seconds, and repeat 3 times.

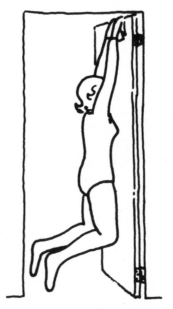

Fig. 18

DOOR STRETCH

Benefits
— Relieves pain of stiff and tense backs.
— Extends the discs.
— Releases tension in spine.
— Increases movement in the lower spine and hip joints.
— Strengthens thighs and legs.

Technique
1. Grab knobs on either side of door at arm's length, feet directly under shoulders.
2. Bend knees slightly, drop head between arms and slowly tuck bottom under and down.
3. Try to lower the buttocks by bending the knees as much as possible. Keep bottom tucked in and lower back rounded throughout.
4. Come out of the pose slowly. Repeat several times.

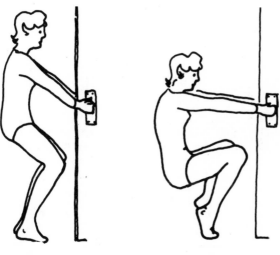

Fig. 19a   Fig. 19b

Variation 1

While in position c, wriggle (wave) your hips gently from side to side.

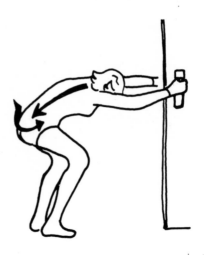

Fig. 19c

Variation 2

Look over your shoulder at your hips as you swivel them. Over left shoulder at left hip, over right shoulder at right hip.

Variation 3

1. Repeat steps 1 and 2, tighten stomach muscles and come slowly up on toes as you go gently down, a little further each day.
2. As you get better, try to force the heels of the feet towards the floor. Rest weight on outside edges, feet well apart.
3. Return slowly to start position. Gradually use only fingertips until you can do the pose standing free.

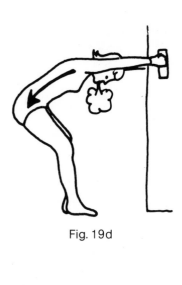

Fig. 19d

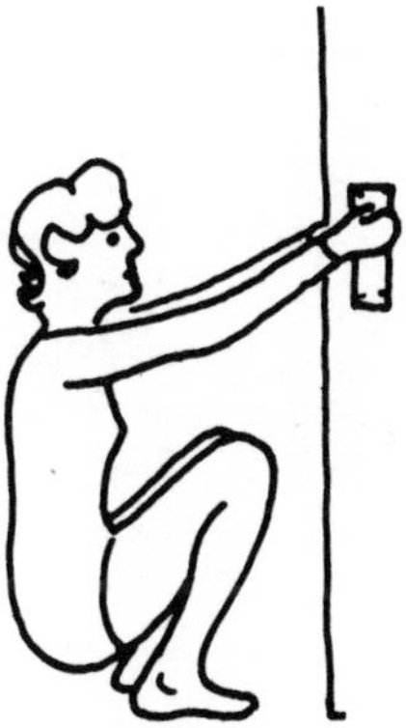

Fig. 19e

KNEE AND THIGH STRETCH

Benefits
— Relieves sciatic pain.

Technique
1. Sit on the floor, legs outstretched, back straight.
2. Bend your knees to the side and bring the soles of your feet together (Figure 20a).
3. Clasp your fingers tightly around the toes and gently pull the feet as close to the body as you can, possibly touching the perineum (Figure 20b).
4. Now with a great effort of will, widen the thighs and attempt to bring the knees to the floor by pulling up on the toes.
5. Hold the position for as long as you can—from 5-30 seconds. The secret here lies in breathing normally as you are holding (Figure 20c).
6. Relax by stretching the legs out and shaking them if you wish.
7. Repeat twice more; or 4 times more if you are really concerned about your health problem or flabby inner thighs.

Dos and Don'ts
— DO clasp your fingers tightly around the toes to give you a good hold and to prevent slipping.
— DON'T push the knees forcibly with your hands. You can accomplish much more by your will.
— DON'T be discouraged if your knees look like craggy mountains for a while. With patient perseverance you have an excellent chance of eventually laying the knees on the floor.
— DO try to relax, even as you are holding.

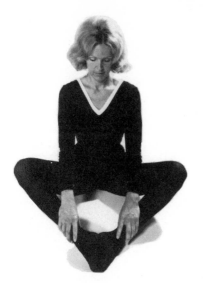

Fig. 20a

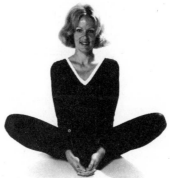

Fig. 20b

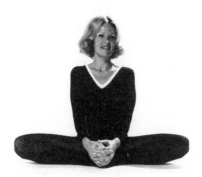

Fig. 20c

KNEE PRESS

Benefits
 — Is recommended for the greatly over-weight and very elderly, because it gives maximum results with a minimum of effort.
 — Relieves backache and strengthens the lumbar region of the back.
 — Strengthens the abdominal muscles.
 — Eases tension in the neck, back and shoulders.
 — Strengthens the neck muscles.

Technique
 1. Lie on your back, legs outstretched, hands by your side.
 2. Bend the right knee and bring it against the chest.
 3. INHALE, clasp your hands around the knee and press it against the abdomen and chest. Keep the left leg straight and the head on the floor.
 4. Hold the pose and your breath for 5-10 seconds (Figure 21a).
 5. EXHALE, lower the leg and relax.
 6. Repeat with the other leg.
 7. Repeat with both legs together.

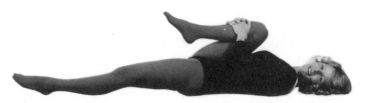

Fig. 21a

Variation
1. Repeat steps 1 and 2 as above.
2. INHALE, clasp your hands around the right knee and press it to the chest.
3. At the same time bring the head up and try to press it to the knee.
4. Hold the pose and your breath for 5-10 seconds (Figure 21b).
5. EXHALE, lower the leg and relax.
6. Repeat on the other side.
7. Repeat with both knees.

Dos and Don'ts
— DON'T hold your breath if you have a record of high blood pressure or heart trouble. Simply inhale and then breathe normally.
— DO keep the knee of the out-stretched leg straight.
— DO get a good grasp on the knees and exert as much pressure as you can on the abdomen.
— DON'T get discouraged if your knee is nowhere near your head at first. The mere effort does wonders for you.

The Knee Press is a 'now' sort of exercise, to be done anytime there is need for it. It relieves, as well as strengthens.

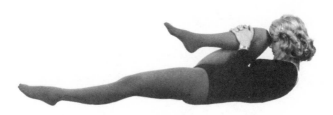

Fig. 21b

LEG-OVER

Benefits
— Relieves sprains in lower back and hip.

Technique
1. Lie on your back, arms stretched out to the side.
2. Lift your right leg slowly until it points straight up. Do not bend the knee throughout (Figure 22a).
3. Move the leg to the left across the body and try to lower it to the floor.
4. Make sure that *both* shoulders stay on the floor, even if you have to grip a chair leg with your right hand.
5. When the leg has gone as far as it will go, turn your head to the right (Figure 22b).
6. Hold the position from 5-20 seconds.
7. Slowly bring the leg up and then lower it.
8. Repeat with the other leg.
9. Then repeat with both legs together (Figure 22c).

Variation
Bend both legs at the knee and bring them to the side.

Dos and Don'ts
— DON'T roll over to the side that your leg is moving to. Keep both shoulders on the floor to give your spine a delightful spiral stretch.
— DO turn your head in the opposite direction of the leg.

The Leg-Over is gentle enough to be safely practised even by the elderly. It gives a maximum stretch to the spine with a minimum of effort.

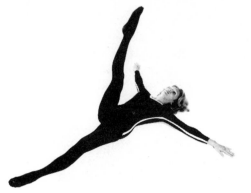

Fig. 22a

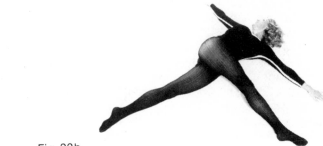

Fig. 22b

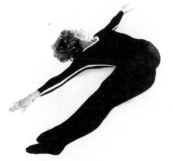

Fig. 22c

LOCUST

Benefits
— Relieves pain in the lumbar and sacral areas of the back and strengthens them.
— Is beneficial to people with slipped disc.
— Improves the circulation to the head for a feeling of alertness and energy.

Technique: The Half Locust
1. Lie on your stomach, hands by your side, palms up.
2. Make a fist and bring it close to the body.
3. Raise your head and bring the front of the chin to the floor.
4. Pressing the arms against the floor, INHALE and slowly raise the right leg straight up in the back as far as you can (Figure 23a).
5. Hold the breath and the pose from 5-10 seconds, EXHALE and slowly lower the leg. Relax.
6. Repeat on the other side, making sure that the body weight is not rolled to the side of the out-stretched leg.
7. As a variation you may make the fists and place them *thumbs* down.

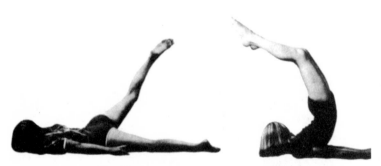

Fig. 23a   Fig. 23b

Technique: The Locust

1. Lie on your stomach, hands by your side palms up.
2. Raise your head and place the front of the chin only, on the floor.
3. Make fists of your hands and place them under the thighs in the groin.
4. INHALE, stiffen the body and pushing down on the arms, bring the legs up as high as they will go (Figures 23b and 23c).
5. Hold the pose for 5-10 seconds, holding breath as well.
6. EXHALE, lower the legs slowly and relax. Rest for a while.

Dos and Don'ts

— DO practice the Half Locust only, for several weeks, to strengthen a weak back.
— DO gather all your energy and concentration on your arms and legs as you inhale in preparation for the Locust.
— DO press your chin firmly into the ground.
— DO try to make your knees as straight as possible.
— DO use great pressure on the arms to raise the legs.
— DO try a slight thrusting movement to get the legs up, *if* you have no record of back problems, and only after a thorough warm-up.
— DO come out of the pose slowly. You nullify a great deal of your effort by collapsing.

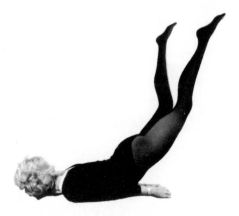

Fig. 23c

PENDULUM

Benefits
— Relieves pain of bursitis.
— Improves circulation to head and upper body.
— Relieves tension and gives a feeling of energy.
— Improves posture.
— Tones muscles of shoulders and upper back.

Technique
1. Stand, feet comfortably apart, your left hand at the waist (Figure 24a).
2. Bend slowly forward from the waist and let the right arm hang limply down.
3. Swing your right arm like a pendulum in a long oval in front of your feet. It is important here that the arm is not stiffly directed by you but swings freely and limply (Figure 24b).
4. Slowly straighten up, bringing the right arm over-head. Stretch it back as far as it will go. Hold. Relax (Figure 24c).
5. Repeat with the other arm.
6. Repeat with both arms.
7. Perform the whole exercise 2-3 times more, reversing the direction of the oval.

Dos and Don'ts
— DO keep the knees straight.
— DON'T move the arm stiffly.

The Pendulum is deceptively simple for people without problems in that area, but for the tense person, or the sufferer of bursitis, this asana gives maximum relief with a minimum of discomfort.

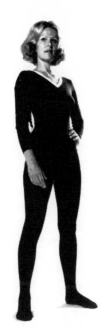

Fig. 24a

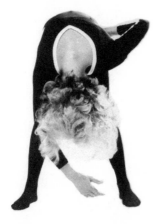

Fig. 24b

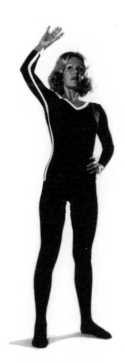

Fig. 24c

REVERSE ARCH

Benefits
— Relieves menstrual and other pains in the lower back.
— Strengthens the sacroiliac region of the back.
— Relieves backache.

Technique
1. Lie on your back, knees bent, feet flat on the floor, arms by your side.
2. Pull the feet as close to the buttocks as possible, without straining.
3. Exhale and slowly tilt the pelvis up, pushing the small of the back against the floor and tightening the muscles of the abdomen and buttocks. The pelvis is NOT lifted, only tilted.
4. Hold the pose, exhale and lower the pelvis. Repeat once more.
5. Now, inhale and slowly push the buttocks and lower body up as high as you can (Figure 25a).
6. Shift the weight towards the shoulders, relax the arms, and breathe normally.
7. Hold 5-30 seconds. Exhale and relax slowly, bringing the back down vertebra by vertebra. Repeat three to four times.

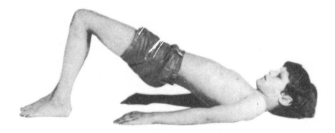

Fig. 25a

Variation 1
1. Repeat steps 1-6.
2. Now, stretch one leg forward. Hold. Relax (Figure 25b).

Variation 2
1. Repeat steps 1-6.
2. Now, come up on your toes and take a step towards the buttocks. Hold. Relax.

Dos and Don'ts
— DO only *tilt* the pelvis without lifting it, in steps 1-4. The buttocks should not be wholly off the floor. The feeling should almost be one of pinching the buttocks together.
— DON'T keep the weight on the arms. Shift the weight to the shoulders and relax the arms as much as possible.
— DO enjoy the delightful stretching sensation in your upper legs.

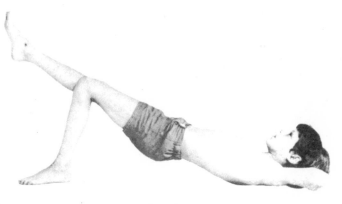

Fig. 25b

ROCK 'N' ROLLS

Benefits
— Act as an excellent warm-up and energizer.
— Limber up the spine.

Technique
1. Sit on the floor, knees bent.
2. Clasp your hands under the knees.
3. Bring your head as close to the knees as possible and keep it there throughout (Figure 26a).
4. Rock gently back onto the spine, keeping the back rounded and the legs together (Figure 26b).
5. Establish an easy rhythm in rocking back and forth (Figure 26c).
6. Repeat 12 times or up to a minute.
7. Remember to breathe.

Dos and Don'ts
— DO start the whole exercise on your back if you are a bit timid about rocking back from a sitting position.
— DO the Rock 'n' Rolls any time you want to get the kinks out of your body.
— DO keep your head close to your knees, to have a rounded spine to rock on.
— DO use the momentum of the first backward rock to return forward again.

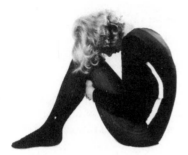

Fig. 26a

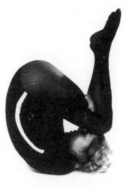

Fig. 26b

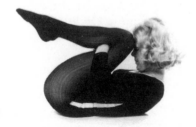

Fig. 26c

SHOULDER-STAND

Benefits
— Improves the circulation to such important areas as the brain, the spine, the pelvic area; these are areas which, due to an upright position, rarely receive a good supply of rich, newly-oxygenated blood.
— Presses the chin against the thryroid gland which stimulates it and reduces excess fat.
— Tones up the central nervous system and soothes it (tension, insomnia) and is a marvellous rejuvenator.
— Has a beneficial effect on the hormone-producing glands of the body.
— Relieves palpitation, breathlessness, bronchitis, throat ailments and asthma due to increased circulation to neck and chest.
— Relieves pressure on abdominal organs due to body-inversion, which, in turn, regulates the digestive processes, frees the body of toxins and increases the energy-level.
— Relieves varicose veins and aching legs.
— Gives new vitality to people who suffer from anaemia or lack of energy.
— Relaxes whole body.
— Stretches the spine.
— Strengthens and firms the muscles of the back, legs, neck and abdomen.

Technique
1. Lie on the floor, legs out-stretched, hands close by your side, palms down.
2. Slowly lift your legs by tensing the abdominal and leg muscles, until they are perpendicular to the floor.
3. Press down on your hands, making them hollow or tent-like (Figure 27a).
4. Raise your buttocks and lower back and grasp yourself around the waist, with the thumbs around the front of the body. DO NOT let the elbows flare out (Figure 27b).
5. Straighten the legs and tuck the bottom in as much as balance permits.
6. If you are balancing well, then grasp yourself up higher on

the rib-cage and tuck your bottom in (Figure 27c).
7. Stretch your legs and point your toes. Hold the position from 10-60 seconds, as a beginner. Gradually work up to 3 minutes. Breathe normally throughout.

Dos and Don'ts

— DO be patient with yourself. The important thing is to be up there at all, even if it is not ramrod-straight at the start.
— DON'T get alarmed if you feel slightly dizzy or heady at first. It is quite normal and can be blamed on the sudden dilation of the blood vessels.

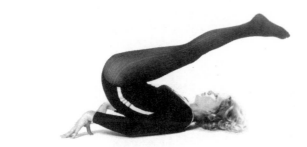

Fig. 27a

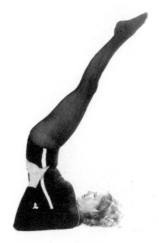

Fig. 27b

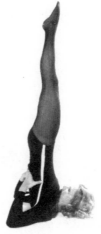

Fig. 27c

SIT-UP

Benefits
— Gently strengthens the back.
— Is one of the best exercises for firming, toning and flattening the abdominal muscles.
— Strengthens and relieves pain in lower back.

Technique
1. Lie on your back, knees bent *just* enough to permit the whole foot to touch the floor.
2. Place your hands on the thighs (Figure 28a).
3. Lift your head slowly and raise your upper body to a 30° angle off the floor, sliding the hands up the legs. Depending on the length of your arms, the fingertips should barely be touching the bent knee-cap.
4. Keeping your back as straight as possible, hold the position 5-30 seconds (Figure 28b).
5. Slowly lower your trunk. Relax.
6. Repeat 3-5 times more.

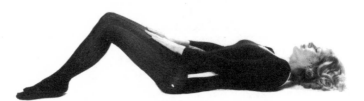

Fig. 28a

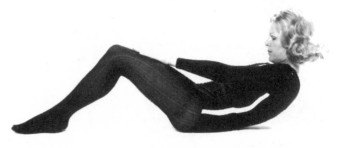

Fig. 28b

Variation 1
1. Follow directions 1 and 2 as above.
2. Lift your upper body slowly, sliding the hands up the legs until you can grasp the knees. Use the knees to pull yourself all the way up (Figure 28c).
3. Slowly return to starting position. Repeat several times.

Variation 2
1. As above.
2. Raise your right shoulder and right knee at the same time and try to bring them together (Figure 28d).
3. Hold, relax. Repeat twice more. Repeat with other leg.

Dos and Don'ts
— DON'T go much further than a 30° angle. If the exercise comes too easily, if the rectal muscles of the abdomen are not standing out in a taut ridge, you may be sure that you are doing it wrong.
— DO breathe normally.

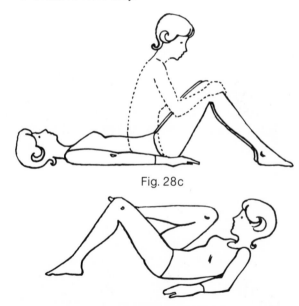

Fig. 28c

Fig. 28d

SPREAD LEG STRETCH

Benefits
— Removes tension of whole body.
— Relieves pains of sciatica.
— Limbers up and makes the spine flexible.

Technique
1. Sit on the floor, legs outstretched and as far apart as possible (Figure 29a).
2. Place your hands on your legs and slowly slide them down toward the toes. Keep the legs straight.
3. Bending forward from the waist, in a curling motion, bring your hands as far as they can go, then grasp that part of the leg you can comfortably reach (Figure 29b).
4. Let your head hang down and bend the elbows to give a good forward stretch. Hold for 10-30 seconds. Relax, slowly return (Figure 29c—advanced pose).
5. Repeat twice more.

Dos and Don'ts
— DO sit well back on your pelvis, not on your tailbone.
— DON'T bend your knees, you will nullify many of the benefits.
— DON'T jerk or bounce.

In the advanced form of this pose, you will be able to lower your head to the floor, which will give you the added benefit of improved circulation to the head.

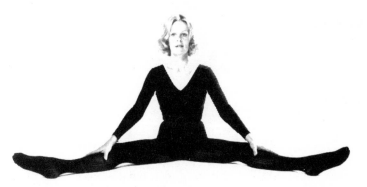

Fig. 29a

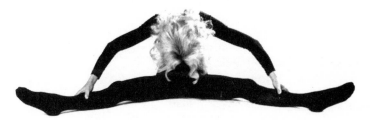

Fig. 29b

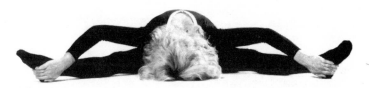

Fig. 29c

STAFF

Benefits
— Promotes poise and grace.
— Strengthens the lower back (especially for elderly people).
— Relieves severe backache.

Technique
1. Sit on your tailbone on the floor, the legs outstretched, the hands by the hips.
2. EXHALE, bend the elbows, lean slightly backward and slowly raise the legs, the knees straight.
3. Concentrate fiercely, as in any balancing exercise, and attempt to bring the feet on a level with the head (Figure 30a).
4. When you have established balance, slowly bring the hands parallel to the floor, the palms facing the legs (Figure 30b).
5. Hold the pose for as long as you can, or 10-30 seconds.
6. The breathing rhythm should be one of INHALE, EXHALE, hold a little, INHALE, etc...
7. EXHALE, lower the legs and relax.

Dos and Don'ts
— DO establish your point of balance by just lifting the feet an inch or two before going into the exercise proper.
— DO hold onto the legs near the knees at first for extra support.
— DO concentrate on your balance—staring at one spot helps.
— DON'T get discouraged if you keep rolling over on your back. Just practise the Tree and other such balancing exercises.

The Staff is an exercise that has benefits for all age groups of both sexes. With the proper breathing it works equally well on the abdominal muscles and abdominal organs, while it strengthens the back as well. In time you will be able to go into it in one fluid motion.

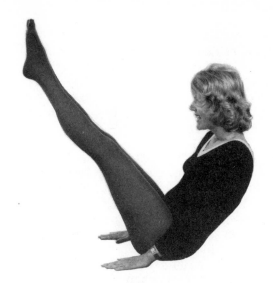

Fig. 30a

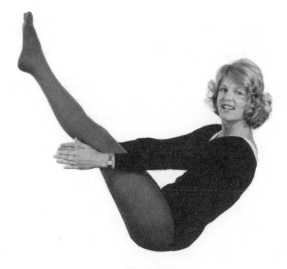

Fig. 30b

TRIANGLE POSTURE

Benefits
— Relieves backache.

Technique
1. Stand with the feet about 36 ins apart.
2. Bring your arms out straight at the sides, parallel to the floor (Figure 31a).
3. Point your right foot 90° outwards, the left foot slightly to the right.
4. Bend your body to the right, bringing the hand as close as possible to the outside of the right foot.
5. Bring your left arm up so that it is in a straight line with the right arm. Look up at the left hand (Figure 31b).
6. Hold 10-30 seconds, breathing normally.
7. Come up slowly.
8. Repeat on the other side.
9. Repeat twice more on each side.

Dos and Don'ts
— DO keep both your knees absolutely straight throughout. It is not so important how far you go as that you do it properly.
— DO stretch your shoulders as you hold.

The Triangle Postures are very reminiscent of calisthenics with the tremendous difference of the tension-dissolving holding action. Try them both and see the difference.

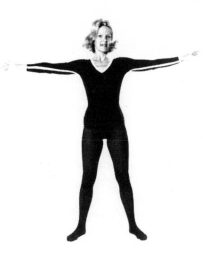

Fig. 31 a

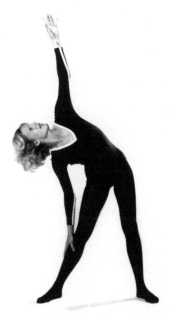

Fig. 31 b

TWIST

Benefits
— Makes spine more supple, which has therapeutic effect on nervous system.
— Realigns vertebrae and relieves tension.

Technique
1. Sit on the floor, legs outstretched.
2. Spread your legs and bring the *right foot* against the *left thigh.* Press the side of the right knee against the floor (Figure 32a).
3. Bend your left knee and, leaving it sticking up in the air, bring the *left foot* over the *right knee* (Figure 32b).
4. Set the sole of the *left foot* squarely on the floor. The further back you can bring the foot, the better.
5. Using both hands for support, shift your weight well forward onto the pelvis, to prevent tipping (Figure 32c).
6. With the *left hand* behind you on the floor for support, raise your *right arm* and bring it between your chest and the left knee (Figure 32d).
7. Twist your body so that your *right shoulder* is resting against the *left knee.*
8. Now make a fist of your *right hand* and move your *right arm* poker-straight over the *right knee* that is lying on the floor.
9. Attempt to get hold of the toes of the left foot. As a beginner, that is nearly impossible, so it is perfectly alright to grasp the right knee.
10. Levering yourself against the *left leg* with the *right arm,* now twist to the left.
11. Bend your left arm and bring the back of the hand against the small of the back.
12. Turn your head to the left and look as far left as you can (Figure 32e).
13. Hold this position for 10-30 seconds.
14. Slowly unwind.
15. Repeat on the other side.

Dos and Don'ts

— DO sit well forward on your pelvis.
— DON'T bend your arm as you draw it across the knee.
— DO swivel your shoulder or upper arm against the knee to permit you to bring your arm around further.

The Twist seems like an almost impossible position to assume at first. A picture here is worth a thousand words. Once you have the idea, however, the Twist will become a most satisfying exercise because it stretches most muscles of the body. The spiral twist that the spine is getting is most beneficial too.

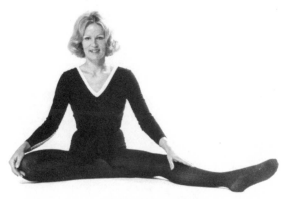

Fig. 32a

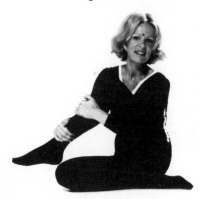

Fig. 32b

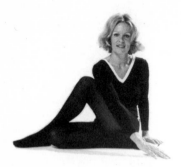

Fig. 32c

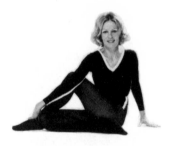

Fig. 32d

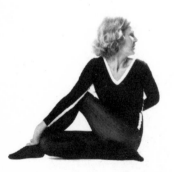

Fig. 32e